Fuel + Fitness 

Hello! CONGRATULATIONS on making the decision to do something new and different to take action on becoming an even better and healthier you! I'm excited to share this simple Fuel + Fitness tracker with you. For years, I struggled with my own weight loss. I tried every fad diet – keto, Atkins, cucumber juicing, fasting – you name it, I tried it. At the age of 40, I began to feel the effects of my unhealthy lifestyle. I was 50 pounds overweight, pre-diabetic, had high blood pressure, and just always felt tired. It really hit me when my husband and I went on vacation to Central America and I nearly fainted during a short hike. There were people twice my age trekking along like it was nothing, and I was on the sidelines barely able to breathe. I couldn't enjoy the beautiful countries we traveled so far to visit because I was so out of shape. And, not to mention, I hated the way I looked in a bathing suit so I couldn't enjoy the beautiful beaches or laying poolside without feeling ashamed. I decided I needed to take serious action to improve my health and self-esteem so that I can really enjoy all that this life and world has to offer.

Through trial and error, I found a routine that worked for me. My goals were to lose 50 pounds and go down 5 sizes. It took me one year to reach my goals. Honestly, as I know with most of you, I was hoping to accomplish my goals much sooner. There were weeks and months when I didn't see much progress on the scale or in the mirror. What I've learned is that even though I didn't see the progress, I was gaining strength, endurance and stamina – all which gave me the ability to push myself harder and break through the plateaus. Most importantly, the year gave me time to settle into my new habits. I've trained myself to view food as fuel to power through the days and workouts. I learned how much and what type of fuel I needed. This wouldn't have happened though without diligent planning and tracking to find what works. I now know what I need to do to keep the weight off and my engine running. Find what works for you. Make a conscious effort to eat healthily, push yourself to your limits during exercise, and track what you're doing in this book so you can make the adjustments and improvements where needed. If you make the effort, I guarantee you'll see positive changes over time.

Here are a few tips that helped me:
1. FOOD IS FUEL. You (only) need enough of the good stuff to get you through your day.
2. Stop drinking soda and juices. Stick to water and unsweetened tea.
3. Limit your added processed sugar intake to a "cheat" snack. But, don't "cheat" at all during the first 30 days so you can truly train yourself.
4. Carbs and starches aren't bad if it isn't processed!
5. Speaking of processed, limit your intake of processed food. That isn't fuel, it's junk. Stick to eating *"real"* whole foods.
6. Learn what a serving size is.
7. All of your meals should be well-rounded to include veggies (mostly), carbs (grains are best) and protein.
8. Exercise for at least 30 minutes every day. Even if it's just stretching or going for a walk during your "rest days".
9. Plan a well-rounded exercise routine to include cardio, strength training and HIIT. And, change up your exercise routine at least every 30 days so you don't plateau. Or, follow a workout program (FitnessBlender or Beachbody has great ones).
10. Don't be afraid to lift heavy weights.
11. You don't have to pay for a gym membership to get a great workout in. YouTube has some great exercise routines you can do at home. My faves are: FitnessBlender, PopSugar Fitness, Yoga with Adriene, Heather Robertson, and Chloe Ting. Even though it's old school, I still love the Beachbody workout programs (including Insanity and P90X).

I am not a fitness or nutrition expert, by no means. I also don't believe that that's what it takes to lose weight or be healthy. IT'S ALL IN YOU. You can be the change you want to see.

Fuel + Fitness

The Before Me

Track where you are now so you can celebrate your progress as you move through this new way of life. Let's create baseline of your weight, measurements, and fitness levels now, and we'll do it again in 30, 60 and 90 days. Try not t do this baseline again before the next 30 days. During this time, your body is in shock with all the changes you're making – you may lose a lot of water weight during the first week and then gain some of that back the following week. You want to give your body some time to adjust and settle into your new habits. That's why it's best to check your progress over time instead of frequently. You will see vast changes, instead of incremental which gives you mo to celebrate!

Current Weight ______________________________

Fit Test	
# of Push Ups	
# of Burpees	
# of Squats	
Plank Hold Time	
1-Mile Run Time	

Measurements			
Chest		Upper Arms (R/L)	
Waist		Thighs (R/L)	
Hips		Calves (R/L)	

Take before and after pictures of yourself at each stage.

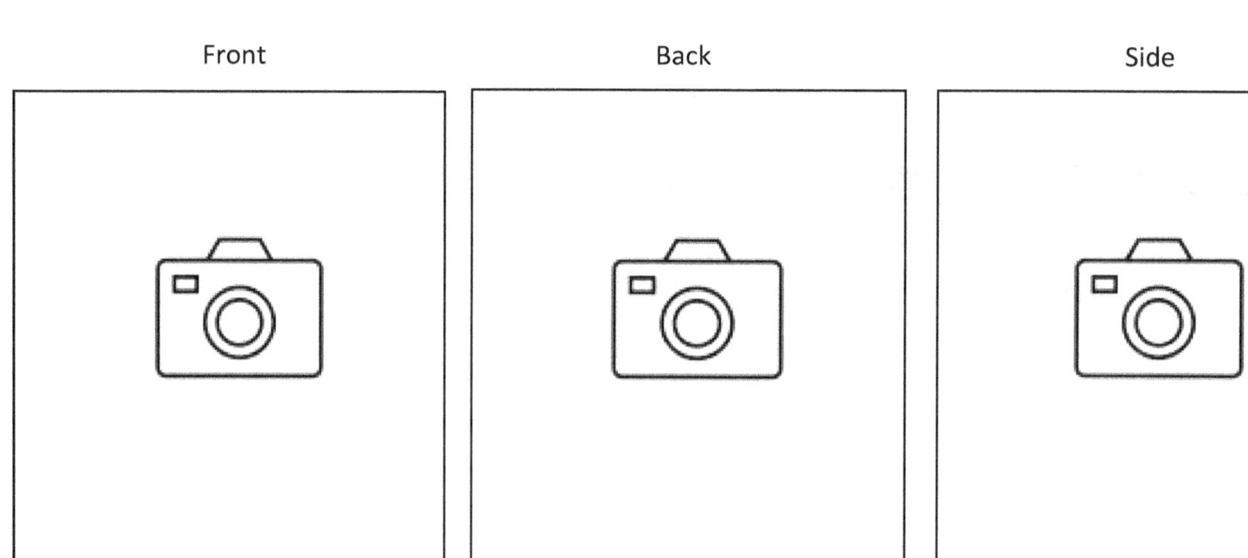

Front Back Side

Fuel + Fitness

Date ______________________

m t w t f s s

Today's Motivation ____

Fuel

Breakfast	
Snack	
Lunch	
Snack	
Dinner	
Notes	

Fitness

Type	Time	Duration	Notes (weights, reps, struggles, etc

Today, I am proud of myself because ____

Tomorrow, I will improve ____

Overall, I felt ____

Fuel + Fitness

Date _________________
m t w t f s s

Today's Motivation ____

Fuel	🍒 🍆 🥜 🍎 🥑 🍌
Breakfast	
Snack	
Lunch	
Snack	
Dinner	
Notes	

Fitness			
Type	Time	Duration	Notes (weights, reps, struggles, etc

Today, I am proud of myself because ____

Tomorrow, I will improve ____

Overall, I felt ____

Fuel + Fitness

Date ___________________

m t w t f s s

Today's Motivation ____

Fuel						
Breakfast						
Snack						
Lunch						
Snack						
Dinner						
Notes						

Fitness			
Type	Time	Duration	Notes (weights, reps, struggles, etc

Today, I am proud of myself because ____

Tomorrow, I will improve ____

Overall, I felt ____

Fuel + Fitness

Date ______________

m t w t f s s

Today's Motivation ____

Fuel						
Breakfast						
Snack						
Lunch						
Snack						
Dinner						
Notes						

Fitness			
Type	Time	Duration	Notes (weights, reps, struggles, etc

Today, I am proud of myself because ____

Tomorrow, I will improve ____

Overall, I felt ____

Fuel + Fitness

Date ______________________

m t w t f s s

Today's Motivation ____

Fuel

Breakfast						
Snack						
Lunch						
Snack						
Dinner						
Notes						

Fitness

Type	Time	Duration	Notes (weights, reps, struggles, etc

Today, I am proud of myself because ____

Tomorrow, I will improve ____

Overall, I felt ____

Fuel + Fitness

Date _______________

m t w t f s s

Today's Motivation ____

Fuel

Breakfast	
Snack	
Lunch	
Snack	
Dinner	
Notes	

Fitness

Type	Time	Duration	Notes (weights, reps, struggles, etc

Today, I am proud of myself because ____

Tomorrow, I will improve ____

Overall, I felt ____

Fuel + Fitness

Date ________________

m t w t f s s

Today's Motivation ____

Fuel

Breakfast	
Snack	
Lunch	
Snack	
Dinner	
Notes	

Fitness

Type	Time	Duration	Notes (weights, reps, struggles, etc

Today, I am proud of myself because ______________________________________

Tomorrow, I will improve ____

Overall, I felt ____

Fuel + Fitness

Date ___________________
m t w t f s s

Today's Motivation ____

Fuel

Breakfast						
Snack						
Lunch						
Snack						
Dinner						
Notes						

Fitness

Type	Time	Duration	Notes (weights, reps, struggles, etc

Today, I am proud of myself because ____

Tomorrow, I will improve ____

Overall, I felt ____

Fuel + Fitness

Date _______________

m t w t f s s

Today's Motivation ____

Fuel						
Breakfast						
Snack						
Lunch						
Snack						
Dinner						
Notes						

Fitness			
Type	Time	Duration	Notes (weights, reps, struggles, etc

Today, I am proud of myself because ____

Tomorrow, I will improve ____

Overall, I felt ____

Fuel + Fitness

Date ________________

m t w t f s s

Today's Motivation ____

Fuel						
Breakfast						
Snack						
Lunch						
Snack						
Dinner						
Notes						

Fitness			
Type	Time	Duration	Notes (weights, reps, struggles, etc

Today, I am proud of myself because ____

Tomorrow, I will improve ____

Overall, I felt ____

Fuel + Fitness

Date _________________

m t w t f s s

Today's Motivation ____

Fuel						
Breakfast						
Snack						
Lunch						
Snack						
Dinner						
Notes						

Fitness			
Type	Time	Duration	Notes (weights, reps, struggles, etc

Today, I am proud of myself because ____

Tomorrow, I will improve ____

Overall, I felt ____

Fuel + Fitness

Date _________________

m t w t f s s

Today's Motivation ____

Fuel						
Breakfast						
Snack						
Lunch						
Snack						
Dinner						
Notes						

Fitness			
Type	Time	Duration	Notes (weights, reps, struggles, etc

Today, I am proud of myself because ____

Tomorrow, I will improve ____

Overall, I felt ____

Fuel + Fitness

Date ___________________

m t w t f s s

Today's Motivation ____

Fuel

Breakfast	
Snack	
Lunch	
Snack	
Dinner	
Notes	

Fitness

Type	Time	Duration	Notes (weights, reps, struggles, etc

Today, I am proud of myself because ____

Tomorrow, I will improve ____

Overall, I felt ____

Fuel + Fitness

Date ___________________

m t w t f s s

Today's Motivation ____

Fuel

Breakfast	
Snack	
Lunch	
Snack	
Dinner	
Notes	

Fitness

Type	Time	Duration	Notes (weights, reps, struggles, etc

Today, I am proud of myself because ____

Tomorrow, I will improve ____

Overall, I felt ____

Fuel + Fitness

Date ___________________

m t w t f s s

Today's Motivation ____

Fuel

Breakfast						
Snack						
Lunch						
Snack						
Dinner						
Notes						

Fitness

Type	Time	Duration	Notes (weights, reps, struggles, etc

Today, I am proud of myself because ____

Tomorrow, I will improve ____

Overall, I felt ____

Fuel + Fitness

Date ________________

m t w t f s s

Today's Motivation ____

Fuel						
Breakfast						
Snack						
Lunch						
Snack						
Dinner						
Notes						

Fitness			
Type	Time	Duration	Notes (weights, reps, struggles, etc

Today, I am proud of myself because ____

Tomorrow, I will improve ____

Overall, I felt ____

Fuel + Fitness

Date ________________

m t w t f s s

Today's Motivation ____

Fuel						
Breakfast						
Snack						
Lunch						
Snack						
Dinner						
Notes						

Fitness			
Type	Time	Duration	Notes (weights, reps, struggles, etc

Today, I am proud of myself because ____

Tomorrow, I will improve ____

Overall, I felt ____

Fuel + Fitness

Date _______________

m t w t f s s

Today's Motivation ____

Fuel						
Breakfast						
Snack						
Lunch						
Snack						
Dinner						
Notes						

Fitness			
Type	Time	Duration	Notes (weights, reps, struggles, etc

Today, I am proud of myself because ____

Tomorrow, I will improve ____

Overall, I felt ____

Fuel + Fitness

Date _______________

m t w t f s s

Today's Motivation ____

Fuel						
Breakfast						
Snack						
Lunch						
Snack						
Dinner						
Notes						

Fitness			
Type	Time	Duration	Notes (weights, reps, struggles, etc

Today, I am proud of myself because ____

Tomorrow, I will improve ____

Overall, I felt ____

Fuel + Fitness

Date ________________

m t w t f s s

Today's Motivation ____

Fuel						
Breakfast						
Snack						
Lunch						
Snack						
Dinner						
Notes						

Fitness			
Type	Time	Duration	Notes (weights, reps, struggles, etc

Today, I am proud of myself because ____

Tomorrow, I will improve ____

Overall, I felt ____

Fuel + Fitness

Date ________________

m t w t f s s

Today's Motivation ____

Fuel

Breakfast	
Snack	
Lunch	
Snack	
Dinner	
Notes	

Fitness

Type	Time	Duration	Notes (weights, reps, struggles, etc

Today, I am proud of myself because ____

Tomorrow, I will improve ____

Overall, I felt ____

Fuel + Fitness

Date ________________

m t w t f s s

Today's Motivation ____

Fuel

Breakfast	
Snack	
Lunch	
Snack	
Dinner	
Notes	

Fitness

Type	Time	Duration	Notes (weights, reps, struggles, etc

Today, I am proud of myself because ____________________________________

Tomorrow, I will improve ____

Overall, I felt ____

Fuel + Fitness

Today's Motivation ____

Fuel	🍒 🍆 🥜 🍎 🥑 🍌
Breakfast	
Snack	
Lunch	
Snack	
Dinner	
Notes	

Fitness			🏋 🤸 🥋 🏊 🧘 🚴
Type	Time	Duration	Notes (weights, reps, struggles, etc

Today, I am proud of myself because _________________________________

Tomorrow, I will improve ____

Overall, I felt ____

Fuel + Fitness

Date ______________

m   t   w   t   f   s   s

Today's Motivation ____

Fuel

Breakfast	
Snack	
Lunch	
Snack	
Dinner	
Notes	

Fitness

Type	Time	Duration	Notes (weights, reps, struggles, etc

Today, I am proud of myself because ____

Tomorrow, I will improve ____

Overall, I felt ____

Fuel + Fitness

Date _______________

m t w t f s s

Today's Motivation ____

Fuel						
Breakfast						
Snack						
Lunch						
Snack						
Dinner						
Notes						

Fitness			
Type	Time	Duration	Notes (weights, reps, struggles, etc

Today, I am proud of myself because ____

Tomorrow, I will improve ____

Overall, I felt ____

Fuel + Fitness

Date ___________________

m t w t f s s

Today's Motivation ____

Fuel						
Breakfast						
Snack						
Lunch						
Snack						
Dinner						
Notes						

Fitness			
Type	Time	Duration	Notes (weights, reps, struggles, etc

Today, I am proud of myself because ____

Tomorrow, I will improve ____

Overall, I felt ____

Fuel + Fitness

Date ________________

m t w t f s s

Today's Motivation ____

Fuel

Breakfast	
Snack	
Lunch	
Snack	
Dinner	
Notes	

Fitness

Type	Time	Duration	Notes (weights, reps, struggles, etc

Today, I am proud of myself because ____

Tomorrow, I will improve ____

Overall, I felt ____

Fuel + Fitness

Today's Motivation ____

Fuel						
Breakfast						
Snack						
Lunch						
Snack						
Dinner						
Notes						

Fitness			
Type	Time	Duration	Notes (weights, reps, struggles, etc

Today, I am proud of myself because ____

Tomorrow, I will improve ____

Overall, I felt ____

Fuel + Fitness

Date ________________

m t w t f s s

Today's Motivation ____

Fuel

Breakfast	
Snack	
Lunch	
Snack	
Dinner	
Notes	

Fitness

Type	Time	Duration	Notes (weights, reps, struggles, etc

Today, I am proud of myself because ____

Tomorrow, I will improve ____

Overall, I felt ____

Fuel + Fitness

Date ________________

m t w t f s s

Today's Motivation ____

Fuel

Breakfast	
Snack	
Lunch	
Snack	
Dinner	
Notes	

Fitness

Type	Time	Duration	Notes (weights, reps, struggles, etc

Today, I am proud of myself because ____

Tomorrow, I will improve ____

Overall, I felt ____

Fuel + Fitness

The **30** Day Me

ongratulations! You made it to day 30! You should be so proud of yourself! Track where you are today, just like you id at the beginning. Use the results to encourage yourself to keep at it. The next 30 days are going to be even better ow that you've established a rhythm!

urrent Weight _________________________________

Fit Test	
# of Push Ups	
# of Burpees	
# of Squats	
Plank Hold Time	
1-Mile Run Time	

Measurements			
Chest		Upper Arms (R/L)	
Waist		Thighs (R/L)	
Hips		Calves (R/L)	

ake before and after pictures of yourself at each stage.

Front	Back	Side
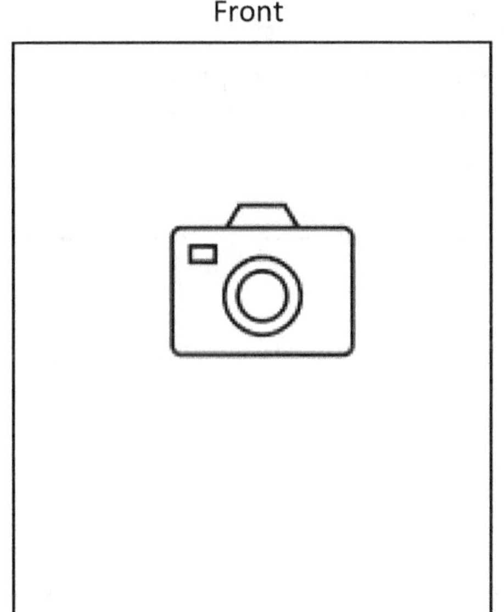	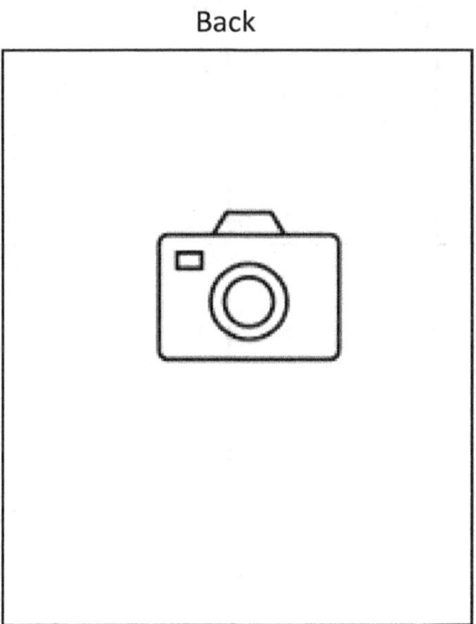	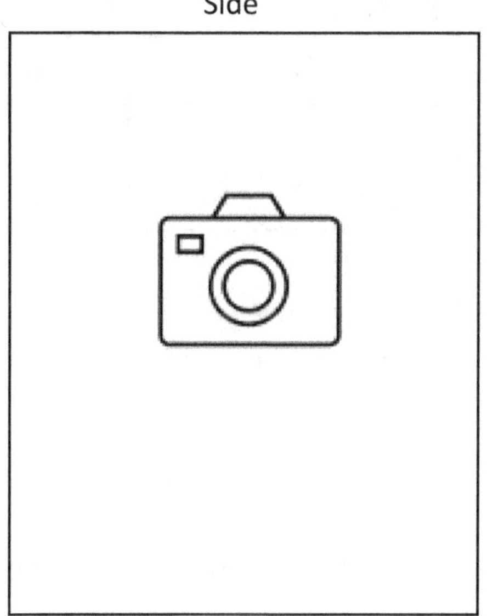

overall, how do you feel? ____

Fuel + Fitness

Date _______________

m t w t f s s

Today's Motivation ____

Fuel						
Breakfast						
Snack						
Lunch						
Snack						
Dinner						
Notes						

Fitness			
Type	Time	Duration	Notes (weights, reps, struggles, etc

Today, I am proud of myself because ____

Tomorrow, I will improve ____

Overall, I felt ____

Fuel + Fitness

Date _______________
m t w t f s s

Today's Motivation ____

Fuel						
Breakfast						
Snack						
Lunch						
Snack						
Dinner						
Notes						

Fitness			
Type	Time	Duration	Notes (weights, reps, struggles, etc

Today, I am proud of myself because ____

Tomorrow, I will improve ____

Overall, I felt ____

Fuel + Fitness

Date _______________

m t w t f s s

Today's Motivation ____

Fuel

Breakfast	
Snack	
Lunch	
Snack	
Dinner	
Notes	

Fitness

Type	Time	Duration	Notes (weights, reps, struggles, etc

Today, I am proud of myself because ____

Tomorrow, I will improve ____

Overall, I felt ____

Fuel + Fitness

Date ________________

m t w t f s s

Today's Motivation ____

Fuel

Breakfast	
Snack	
Lunch	
Snack	
Dinner	
Notes	

Fitness

Type	Time	Duration	Notes (weights, reps, struggles, etc

Today, I am proud of myself because ____

Tomorrow, I will improve ____

Overall, I felt ____

Fuel + Fitness

Date ______________

m t w t f s s

Today's Motivation ____

Fuel						
Breakfast						
Snack						
Lunch						
Snack						
Dinner						
Notes						

Fitness			
Type	Time	Duration	Notes (weights, reps, struggles, etc

Today, I am proud of myself because ____

Tomorrow, I will improve ____

Overall, I felt ____

Fuel + Fitness

Date ___________________

m t w t f s s

Today's Motivation ____

Fuel						
Breakfast						
Snack						
Lunch						
Snack						
Dinner						
Notes						

Fitness			
Type	Time	Duration	Notes (weights, reps, struggles, etc

Today, I am proud of myself because ____

Tomorrow, I will improve ____

Overall, I felt ____

Fuel + Fitness

Date __________________

m t w t f s s

Today's Motivation ____

Fuel

Breakfast	
Snack	
Lunch	
Snack	
Dinner	
Notes	

Fitness

Type	Time	Duration	Notes (weights, reps, struggles, etc

Today, I am proud of myself because ____

Tomorrow, I will improve ____

Overall, I felt ____

Fuel + Fitness

Date ___________________

m t w t f s s

Today's Motivation ____

Fuel

Fuel						
Breakfast						
Snack						
Lunch						
Snack						
Dinner						
Notes						

Fitness

Type	Time	Duration	Notes (weights, reps, struggles, etc

Today, I am proud of myself because ____

Tomorrow, I will improve ____

Overall, I felt ____

Fuel + Fitness

Date ______________________

m t w t f s s

Today's Motivation ____

Fuel

Breakfast	
Snack	
Lunch	
Snack	
Dinner	
Notes	

Fitness

Type	Time	Duration	Notes (weights, reps, struggles, etc

Today, I am proud of myself because ______________________________________

Tomorrow, I will improve ______________________________________

Overall, I felt ______________________________________

Fuel + Fitness

Date ________________

m t w t f s s

Today's Motivation ____

Fuel	
Breakfast	
Snack	
Lunch	
Snack	
Dinner	
Notes	

Fitness			
Type	Time	Duration	Notes (weights, reps, struggles, etc

Today, I am proud of myself because ____

Tomorrow, I will improve ____

Overall, I felt ____

Fuel + Fitness

Date ___________________

m t w t f s s

Today's Motivation ____

Fuel						
Breakfast						
Snack						
Lunch						
Snack						
Dinner						
Notes						

Fitness			
Type	Time	Duration	Notes (weights, reps, struggles, etc

Today, I am proud of myself because ____

Tomorrow, I will improve ____

Overall, I felt ____

Fuel + Fitness

Date ________________

m t w t f s s

Today's Motivation ____

Fuel						
Breakfast						
Snack						
Lunch						
Snack						
Dinner						
Notes						

Fitness			
Type	Time	Duration	Notes (weights, reps, struggles, etc

Today, I am proud of myself because ____

Tomorrow, I will improve ____

Overall, I felt ____

Fuel + Fitness

Date ______________
m t w t f s s

Today's Motivation ____

Fuel						
Breakfast						
Snack						
Lunch						
Snack						
Dinner						
Notes						

Fitness			
Type	Time	Duration	Notes (weights, reps, struggles, etc

Today, I am proud of myself because ____

Tomorrow, I will improve ____

Overall, I felt ____

Fuel + Fitness

Date ________________
m t w t f s s

Today's Motivation ____

Fuel	
Breakfast	
Snack	
Lunch	
Snack	
Dinner	
Notes	

Fitness			
Type	Time	Duration	Notes (weights, reps, struggles, etc

Today, I am proud of myself because ____

Tomorrow, I will improve ____

Overall, I felt ____

Fuel + Fitness

Date ________________

m t w t f s s

Today's Motivation ____

Fuel

Breakfast	
Snack	
Lunch	
Snack	
Dinner	
Notes	

Fitness

Type	Time	Duration	Notes (weights, reps, struggles, etc

Today, I am proud of myself because ____

Tomorrow, I will improve ____

Overall, I felt ____

Fuel + Fitness

Date ________________

m t w t f s s

Today's Motivation ____

Fuel

Breakfast	
Snack	
Lunch	
Snack	
Dinner	
Notes	

Fitness

Type	Time	Duration	Notes (weights, reps, struggles, etc

Today, I am proud of myself because ______________________________________

Tomorrow, I will improve ____

Overall, I felt ____

Fuel + Fitness

Date ________________

m t w t f s s

Today's Motivation ____

Fuel	
Breakfast	
Snack	
Lunch	
Snack	
Dinner	
Notes	

Fitness			
Type	Time	Duration	Notes (weights, reps, struggles, etc

Today, I am proud of myself because ____

Tomorrow, I will improve ____

Overall, I felt ____

Fuel + Fitness

Date ______________________

m t w t f s s

Today's Motivation ____

Fuel						
Breakfast						
Snack						
Lunch						
Snack						
Dinner						
Notes						

Fitness			
Type	Time	Duration	Notes (weights, reps, struggles, etc

Today, I am proud of myself because ____

Tomorrow, I will improve ____

Overall, I felt ____

Fuel + Fitness

Date ___________________
m t w t f s s

Today's Motivation ____

Fuel

Breakfast						
Snack						
Lunch						
Snack						
Dinner						
Notes						

Fitness

Type	Time	Duration	Notes (weights, reps, struggles, etc

Today, I am proud of myself because ____

Tomorrow, I will improve ____

Overall, I felt ____

Fuel + Fitness

Date _________________________

m t w t f s s

Today's Motivation ____

Fuel						
Breakfast						
Snack						
Lunch						
Snack						
Dinner						
Notes						

Fitness			
Type	Time	Duration	Notes (weights, reps, struggles, etc

Today, I am proud of myself because ____

Tomorrow, I will improve ____

Overall, I felt ____

Fuel + Fitness

Date ________________

m t w t f s s

Today's Motivation ____

Fuel						
Breakfast						
Snack						
Lunch						
Snack						
Dinner						
Notes						

Fitness			
Type	Time	Duration	Notes (weights, reps, struggles, etc

Today, I am proud of myself because ____

Tomorrow, I will improve ____

Overall, I felt ____

Fuel + Fitness

Date ______________________

m t w t f s s

Today's Motivation ____

Fuel						
Breakfast						
Snack						
Lunch						
Snack						
Dinner						
Notes						

Fitness			
Type	Time	Duration	Notes (weights, reps, struggles, etc

Today, I am proud of myself because ____

Tomorrow, I will improve ____

Overall, I felt ____

Fuel + Fitness

Date ________________

m t w t f s s

Today's Motivation ____

Fuel

Breakfast	
Snack	
Lunch	
Snack	
Dinner	
Notes	

Fitness

Type	Time	Duration	Notes (weights, reps, struggles, etc

Today, I am proud of myself because ____

Tomorrow, I will improve ____

Overall, I felt ____

Fuel + Fitness

Date _______________

m t w t f s s

Today's Motivation ____

Fuel

Breakfast	
Snack	
Lunch	
Snack	
Dinner	
Notes	

Fitness

Type	Time	Duration	Notes (weights, reps, struggles, etc

Today, I am proud of myself because ____

Tomorrow, I will improve ____

Overall, I felt ____

Fuel + Fitness

Date _______________

m t w t f s s

Today's Motivation ____

Fuel						
Breakfast						
Snack						
Lunch						
Snack						
Dinner						
Notes						

Fitness			
Type	Time	Duration	Notes (weights, reps, struggles, etc

Today, I am proud of myself because ____

Tomorrow, I will improve ____

Overall, I felt ____

Fuel + Fitness

Date ________________

m t w t f s s

Today's Motivation ____

Fuel						
Breakfast						
Snack						
Lunch						
Snack						
Dinner						
Notes						

Fitness			
Type	Time	Duration	Notes (weights, reps, struggles, etc

Today, I am proud of myself because ____

Tomorrow, I will improve ____

Overall, I felt ____

Fuel + Fitness

Date ________________

m t w t f s s

Today's Motivation ____

Fuel

Breakfast	
Snack	
Lunch	
Snack	
Dinner	
Notes	

Fitness

Type	Time	Duration	Notes (weights, reps, struggles, etc

Today, I am proud of myself because ____________________________________

Tomorrow, I will improve ____

Overall, I felt ____

Fuel + Fitness

Date _______________

m t w t f s s

Today's Motivation ____

Fuel

Breakfast	
Snack	
Lunch	
Snack	
Dinner	
Notes	

Fitness

Type	Time	Duration	Notes (weights, reps, struggles, etc

Today, I am proud of myself because ____

Tomorrow, I will improve ____

Overall, I felt ____

Fuel + Fitness

Date _______________

m t w t f s s

Today's Motivation ____

Fuel						
Breakfast						
Snack						
Lunch						
Snack						
Dinner						
Notes						

Fitness			
Type	Time	Duration	Notes (weights, reps, struggles, etc

Today, I am proud of myself because ____

Tomorrow, I will improve ____

Overall, I felt ____

Fuel + Fitness

Date ______________________
m t w t f s s

Today's Motivation ____

Fuel						
Breakfast						
Snack						
Lunch						
Snack						
Dinner						
Notes						

Fitness

Type	Time	Duration	Notes (weights, reps, struggles, etc

Today, I am proud of myself because ______________________________________

Tomorrow, I will improve ____

Overall, I felt ____

Fuel + Fitness

The **60** Day Me

Congratulations! You made it to day 60! That is 60 days of determination and showing up for yourself. Again, you should be proud. By now, you should notice positive changes with your body and fitness level. Let's keep this momentum going for another 30 days!

Current Weight ________________________

Fit Test	
# of Push Ups	
# of Burpees	
# of Squats	
Plank Hold Time	
1-Mile Run Time	

Measurements			
Chest		Upper Arms (R/L)	
Waist		Thighs (R/L)	
Hips		Calves (R/L)	

Take before and after pictures of yourself at each stage.

Front	Back	Side
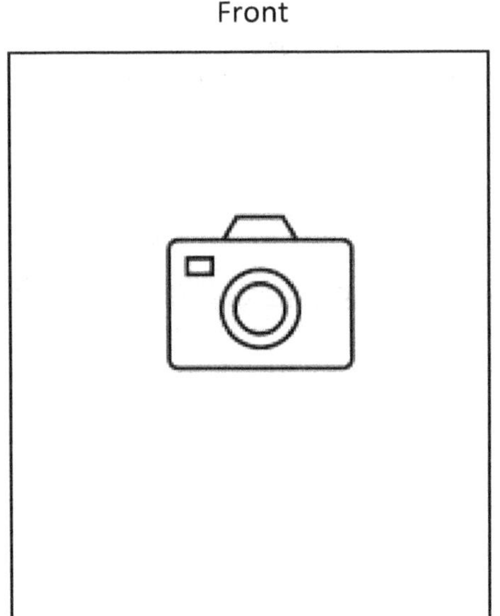	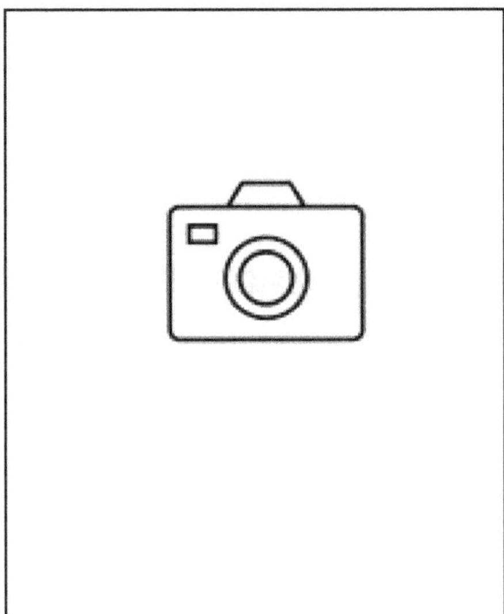	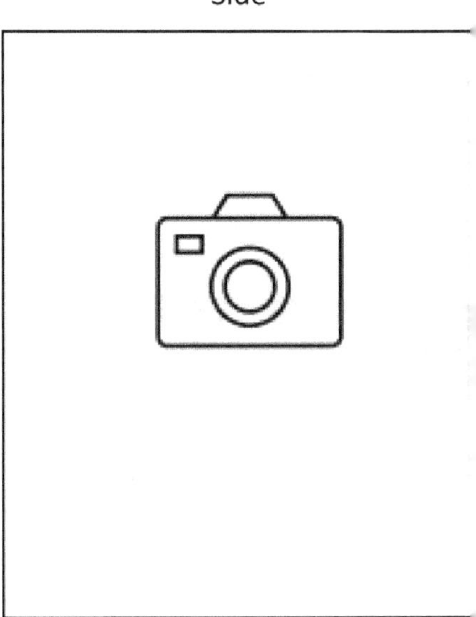

Overall, how do you feel? ____

Fuel + Fitness

Date ___________________

m t w t f s s

Today's Motivation ____

Fuel

Breakfast	
Snack	
Lunch	
Snack	
Dinner	
Notes	

Fitness

Type	Time	Duration	Notes (weights, reps, struggles, etc

Today, I am proud of myself because ____

Tomorrow, I will improve ____

Overall, I felt ____

Fuel + Fitness

Date ________________

m t w t f s s

Today's Motivation ____

Fuel						
Breakfast						
Snack						
Lunch						
Snack						
Dinner						
Notes						

Fitness			
Type	Time	Duration	Notes (weights, reps, struggles, etc

Today, I am proud of myself because ____

Tomorrow, I will improve ____

Overall, I felt ____

Fuel + Fitness

Date ________________

m t w t f s s

Today's Motivation ____

Fuel

Breakfast	
Snack	
Lunch	
Snack	
Dinner	
Notes	

Fitness

Type	Time	Duration	Notes (weights, reps, struggles, etc

Today, I am proud of myself because ____

Tomorrow, I will improve ____

Overall, I felt ____

Fuel + Fitness

Date ________________

m t w t f s s

Today's Motivation ____

Fuel	
Breakfast	
Snack	
Lunch	
Snack	
Dinner	
Notes	

Fitness			
Type	Time	Duration	Notes (weights, reps, struggles, etc

Today, I am proud of myself because ____

Tomorrow, I will improve ____

Overall, I felt ____

Fuel + Fitness

Date ______________________

m   t   w   t   f   s   s

Today's Motivation ____

Fuel						
Breakfast						
Snack						
Lunch						
Snack						
Dinner						
Notes						

Fitness			
Type	Time	Duration	Notes (weights, reps, struggles, etc

Today, I am proud of myself because _______________________________________

Tomorrow, I will improve ____

Overall, I felt ____

Fuel + Fitness

Date ______________________

m t w t f s s

Today's Motivation ____

Fuel						
Breakfast						
Snack						
Lunch						
Snack						
Dinner						
Notes						

Fitness			
Type	Time	Duration	Notes (weights, reps, struggles, etc

Today, I am proud of myself because ______________________________________

Tomorrow, I will improve ______________________________________

Overall, I felt ______________________________________

Fuel + Fitness

Date ________________

m t w t f s s

Today's Motivation ____

Fuel						
Breakfast						
Snack						
Lunch						
Snack						
Dinner						
Notes						

Fitness			
Type	Time	Duration	Notes (weights, reps, struggles, etc

Today, I am proud of myself because ____

Tomorrow, I will improve ____

Overall, I felt ____

Fuel + Fitness

Date ________________

m t w t f s s

Today's Motivation ____

Fuel

Fuel	
Breakfast	
Snack	
Lunch	
Snack	
Dinner	
Notes	

Fitness

Type	Time	Duration	Notes (weights, reps, struggles, etc

Today, I am proud of myself because ____

Tomorrow, I will improve ____

Overall, I felt ____

Fuel + Fitness

Date ________________

m t w t f s s

Today's Motivation ____

Fuel

Breakfast	
Snack	
Lunch	
Snack	
Dinner	
Notes	

Fitness

Type	Time	Duration	Notes (weights, reps, struggles, etc

Today, I am proud of myself because ____

Tomorrow, I will improve ____

Overall, I felt ____

Fuel + Fitness

Date ________________

m t w t f s s

Today's Motivation ____

Fuel

Breakfast	
Snack	
Lunch	
Snack	
Dinner	
Notes	

Fitness

Type	Time	Duration	Notes (weights, reps, struggles, etc

Today, I am proud of myself because ____

Tomorrow, I will improve ____

Overall, I felt ____

Fuel + Fitness

Date ________________

m t w t f s s

Today's Motivation ____

Fuel						
Breakfast						
Snack						
Lunch						
Snack						
Dinner						
Notes						

Fitness			
Type	Time	Duration	Notes (weights, reps, struggles, etc

Today, I am proud of myself because ____

Tomorrow, I will improve ____

Overall, I felt ____

Fuel + Fitness

Date ________________

m t w t f s s

Today's Motivation ____

Fuel						
Breakfast						
Snack						
Lunch						
Snack						
Dinner						
Notes						

Fitness			
Type	Time	Duration	Notes (weights, reps, struggles, etc

Today, I am proud of myself because ____

Tomorrow, I will improve ____

Overall, I felt ____

Fuel + Fitness

Date ________________

m t w t f s s

Today's Motivation ____

Fuel

Breakfast	
Snack	
Lunch	
Snack	
Dinner	
Notes	

Fitness

Type	Time	Duration	Notes (weights, reps, struggles, etc

Today, I am proud of myself because ____

Tomorrow, I will improve ____

Overall, I felt ____

Fuel + Fitness

Date __________________

m t w t f s s

Today's Motivation ____

Fuel

Breakfast	
Snack	
Lunch	
Snack	
Dinner	
Notes	

Fitness

Type	Time	Duration	Notes (weights, reps, struggles, etc

Today, I am proud of myself because ____

Tomorrow, I will improve ____

Overall, I felt ____

Fuel + Fitness

Date ____________________

m t w t f s s

Today's Motivation ____

Fuel

Breakfast						
Snack						
Lunch						
Snack						
Dinner						
Notes						

Fitness

Type	Time	Duration	Notes (weights, reps, struggles, etc

Today, I am proud of myself because ____

Tomorrow, I will improve ____

Overall, I felt ____

Fuel + Fitness

Date ______________

m t w t f s s

Today's Motivation ____

Fuel

Breakfast	
Snack	
Lunch	
Snack	
Dinner	
Notes	

Fitness

Type	Time	Duration	Notes (weights, reps, struggles, etc

Today, I am proud of myself because ____

Tomorrow, I will improve ____

Overall, I felt ____

Fuel + Fitness

Date _______________

m t w t f s s

Today's Motivation ____

Fuel

Breakfast	
Snack	
Lunch	
Snack	
Dinner	
Notes	

Fitness

Type	Time	Duration	Notes (weights, reps, struggles, etc

Today, I am proud of myself because ____

Tomorrow, I will improve ____

Overall, I felt ____

Fuel + Fitness

Date _______________

m t w t f s s

Today's Motivation ____

Fuel						
Breakfast						
Snack						
Lunch						
Snack						
Dinner						
Notes						

Fitness			
Type	Time	Duration	Notes (weights, reps, struggles, etc

Today, I am proud of myself because _______________________________________

Tomorrow, I will improve _______________________________________

Overall, I felt _______________________________________

Fuel + Fitness

Date ________________

m t w t f s s

Today's Motivation ____

Fuel						
Breakfast						
Snack						
Lunch						
Snack						
Dinner						
Notes						

Fitness			
Type	Time	Duration	Notes (weights, reps, struggles, etc

Today, I am proud of myself because ____

Tomorrow, I will improve ____

Overall, I felt ____

Fuel + Fitness

Date ________________

m t w t f s s

Today's Motivation ____

Fuel

Breakfast	
Snack	
Lunch	
Snack	
Dinner	
Notes	

Fitness

Type	Time	Duration	Notes (weights, reps, struggles, etc

Today, I am proud of myself because ____

Tomorrow, I will improve ____

Overall, I felt ____

Fuel + Fitness

Date ___________________

m t w t f s s

Today's Motivation ____

Fuel

Breakfast						
Snack						
Lunch						
Snack						
Dinner						
Notes						

Fitness

Type	Time	Duration	Notes (weights, reps, struggles, etc

Today, I am proud of myself because ____

Tomorrow, I will improve ____

Overall, I felt ____

Fuel + Fitness

Date ________________

m t w t f s s

Today's Motivation ____

Fuel

Breakfast	
Snack	
Lunch	
Snack	
Dinner	
Notes	

Fitness

Type	Time	Duration	Notes (weights, reps, struggles, etc

Today, I am proud of myself because ____

Tomorrow, I will improve ____

Overall, I felt ____

Fuel + Fitness

Date ___________________

Today's Motivation ____

Fuel

Breakfast						
Snack						
Lunch						
Snack						
Dinner						
Notes						

Fitness

Type	Time	Duration	Notes (weights, reps, struggles, etc

Today, I am proud of myself because ____

Tomorrow, I will improve ____

Overall, I felt ____

Fuel + Fitness

Date ________________

m t w t f s s

Today's Motivation ____

Fuel						
Breakfast						
Snack						
Lunch						
Snack						
Dinner						
Notes						

Fitness			
Type	Time	Duration	Notes (weights, reps, struggles, etc

Today, I am proud of myself because ____

Tomorrow, I will improve ____

Overall, I felt ____

Fuel + Fitness

Date ________________

m t w t f s s

Today's Motivation ____

Fuel

Breakfast	
Snack	
Lunch	
Snack	
Dinner	
Notes	

Fitness

Type	Time	Duration	Notes (weights, reps, struggles, etc

Today, I am proud of myself because ____

Tomorrow, I will improve ____

Overall, I felt ____

Fuel + Fitness

Date ______________________

m t w t f s s

Today's Motivation ____

Fuel						
Breakfast						
Snack						
Lunch						
Snack						
Dinner						
Notes						

Fitness			
Type	Time	Duration	Notes (weights, reps, struggles, etc

Today, I am proud of myself because ____________________________________

Tomorrow, I will improve ____________________________________

Overall, I felt ____________________________________

Fuel + Fitness

Date ________________
m t w t f s s

Today's Motivation ____

Fuel

Breakfast	
Snack	
Lunch	
Snack	
Dinner	
Notes	

Fitness

Type	Time	Duration	Notes (weights, reps, struggles, etc

Today, I am proud of myself because ____

Tomorrow, I will improve ____

Overall, I felt ____

Fuel + Fitness

Date ________________

m t w t f s s

Today's Motivation ____

Fuel						
Breakfast						
Snack						
Lunch						
Snack						
Dinner						
Notes						

Fitness			
Type	Time	Duration	Notes (weights, reps, struggles, etc

Today, I am proud of myself because ____

Tomorrow, I will improve ____

Overall, I felt ____

Fuel + Fitness

Date _______________

m t w t f s s

Today's Motivation ____

Fuel						
Breakfast						
Snack						
Lunch						
Snack						
Dinner						
Notes						

Fitness			
Type	Time	Duration	Notes (weights, reps, struggles, etc

Today, I am proud of myself because ____

Tomorrow, I will improve ____

Overall, I felt ____

Fuel + Fitness

Date _______________

m t w t f s s

Today's Motivation ____

Fuel

Breakfast	
Snack	
Lunch	
Snack	
Dinner	
Notes	

Fitness

Type	Time	Duration	Notes (weights, reps, struggles, etc

Today, I am proud of myself because ____

Tomorrow, I will improve ____

Overall, I felt ____

Fuel + Fitness

Date _________________________

m t w t f s s

The 90 Day Me

Congratulations! You've made it to the end of this book. No matter what your results are below, be proud of the commitment you've made to becoming a better you. You've worked hard, challenged yourself and made better decisions for your health.

Current Weight _____________________________

Fit Test	
# of Push Ups	
# of Burpees	
# of Squats	
Plank Hold Time	
1-Mile Run Time	

Measurements			
Chest		Upper Arms (R/L)	
Waist		Thighs (R/L)	
Hips		Calves (R/L)	

Take before and after pictures of yourself at each stage.

Front	Back	Side
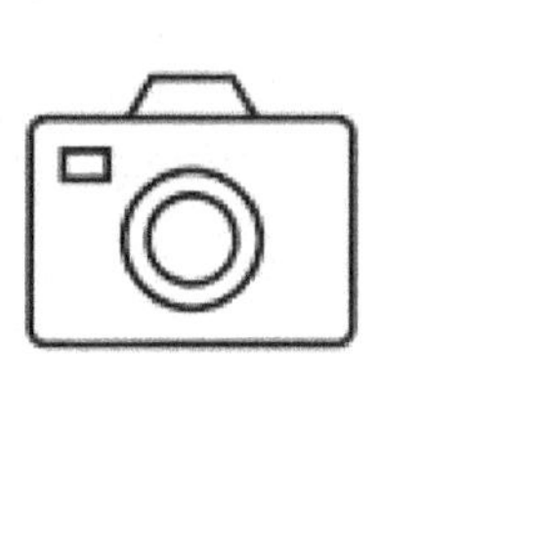	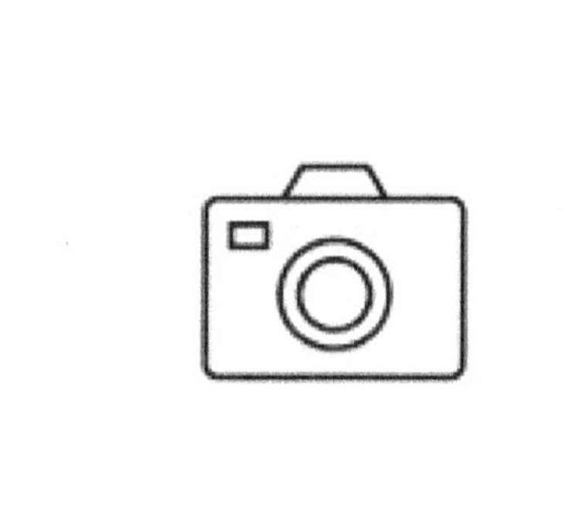	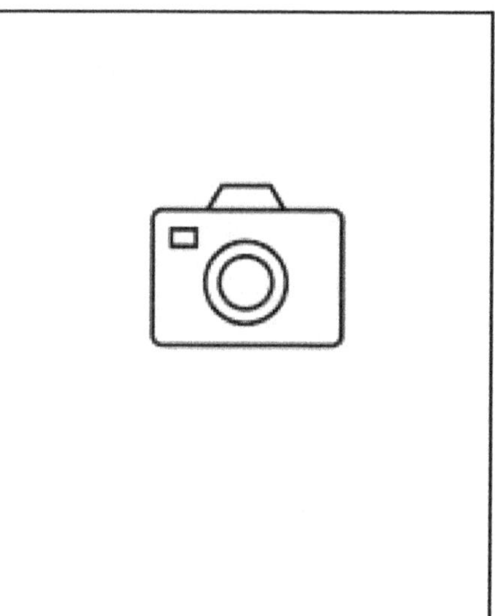

Overall, how do you feel? ____

Fuel + Fitness

Now that you've completed this book, what's next? You've built the foundation to keep your healthy routine going. This is a lifestyle change and you don't want to revert to your old habits. You know what works for you – you know what to do to get or keep the weight off, to stay energized and feeling good. You don't necessarily need to continue tracking your progress now that you've established your routine. Just stick to it. Stay disciplined and committed to continuously improving yourself. Set challenging goals and work hard towards them. Make it fun – try new healthy recipes and new workouts. Just don't give up. You've committed the past 90 days to living better so you know you have it in you to KEEP IT GOING.

I have found that getting others involved in this healthy lifestyle change is a great way to make real sustaining change. Your results will inspire others, and they will look to you for motivation and tips. You will start to feel some responsibility to be a role model ("practice what you a preach") and for their success. Additionally, as you start to check-in on their progress, you establish accountability on both your part and theirs. And last but certainly not least, it's fun! Especially when you can challenge and compete with each other during workouts.

I hope you found this book helpful. My main goal for creating this book was to share what works for me, and help others find what works for them. We all deserve to live the life we imagine for ourselves and it's up to us to make it happen. Fuel yourself with love so that you have the energy to live your best life.

Enjoy the journey!